100 FOODS

BEFORE ONE YEAR

Print ISBN: 978-1-63616-160-0

Published & Illustarted By Opportune Independent Publishing Company

Disclaimer

The information provided in 100 Foods Before One Year is intended for general guidance and informational purposes only. While every effort has been made to ensure the accuracy and reliability of the content, it should not be considered a substitute for professional medical advice, diagnosis, or treatment.

This book is not a replacement for personalized advice from a qualified healthcare provider, pediatrician, or allergist. Every baby is unique, and individual dietary needs and considerations may vary. Readers are strongly encouraged to consult with a healthcare professional before making any decisions related to their baby's nutrition, allergies, or dietary choices.

The author, publisher, and contributors of this book disclaim any liability for any adverse effects or consequences resulting from the use or interpretation of the information presented herein. The book's content is subject to change as new research and medical guidelines emerge, and readers are advised to stay informed of the latest developments in pediatric nutrition and allergies.

Readers should exercise their discretion and judgment when implementing any recommendations or advice provided in this book, taking into consideration their baby's specific health status, allergies, and individual circumstances. It is essential to prioritize the safety and well-being of your child in all dietary and medical decisions.

By using this book, readers acknowledge and accept the terms of this disclaimer and agree to consult with healthcare professionals for personalized guidance on their baby's nutritional and allergy-related needs.

INTRODUCTION

WHAT THIS BOOK CAN BE USED FOR AND HOW TO USE IT

Welcome to *100 Foods Before One Year*! This book is your passport to an incredible journey of introducing your precious little one to the wide and wonderful world of solid foods.

Parenthood is a remarkable adventure filled with countless milestones, and one of the most exciting and memorable moments is the transition to solid foods. It's a time when your baby takes their very first bites, exploring new flavors, textures, and tastes. But with this exciting stage comes a myriad of questions and decisions. What foods should you introduce first? How can you ensure your baby's safety when exploring unfamiliar foods? What about allergies?

100 Foods Before One Year is here to be your trusted companion throughout this adventure. This journaling guide is designed to offer invaluable support and guidance for parents like you, empowering you to make informed decisions about your baby's diet while making the process enjoyable and stress-free.

HOW TO MAKE THE MOST OF THIS BOOK

Discover 100 Foods: Discover 100 Foods: Inside these pages, you'll find detailed profiles of 100 diverse foods, ranging from fruits and vegetables to grains and proteins. These profiles provide essential information on each food's nutritional value and offer tips on how to prepare and introduce them to your baby.

Navigate Allergies with Confidence: We understand that allergies can be a concern for many parents. Our guide includes comprehensive information on common allergens and how to introduce them safely, helping you make informed choices while keeping your baby's health a top priority.

Track Your Baby's Journey: Use the included tracking templates to record your baby's food preferences, reactions, and developmental milestones. This journaling aspect of the book will not only help you keep a detailed record of your baby's culinary adventure but also create beautiful memories to cherish.

Baby-Led Weaning Support: If you're interested in baby-led weaning, our guide provides a comprehensive overview of this approach, including age-appropriate foods and safety precautions.

Parenthood is a unique and extraordinary journey, and 100 Foods Before One Year is here to support you every step of the way. Whether you're a first-time parent or simply seeking fresh insights, this book will help you create a nourishing and positive food experience for your baby. So, open these pages, embrace the adventure, and savor the joy of watching your little one discover the delightful world of food—one bite at a time.

WHO CAN USE IT

Whether you're a first-time parent filled with anticipation and questions or a seasoned caregiver seeking fresh insights, this book is crafted to cater to a wide audience. Here's who can benefit from the invaluable information within these pages:

First-Time Parents: If you're a first-time parent, the world of introducing solid foods to your baby can seem both thrilling and daunting. *100 Foods Before One Year* offers you a reliable roadmap, taking you step by step through the process and helping you make informed choices for your baby's early nutrition.

Experienced Caregivers: Even if you've been through this journey before, each child is unique. This guide equips experienced caregivers with updated information on food introductions, allergies, and baby-led weaning, ensuring you're up to date with the latest practices.

Parents with Allergy Concerns:For parents with concerns about food allergies or a family history of allergies, this book provides essential guidance on identifying potential allergens and safely introducing them into your baby's diet.

Baby-Led Weaning Enthusiasts: If you're interested in exploring the world of baby-led weaning, *100 Foods Before One Year* offers a comprehensive section dedicated to this approach, with practical advice and age-appropriate food options.

Anyone Seeking Nutritional Insights: Beyond the basics, this book offers detailed profiles of 100 foods, shedding light on their nutritional benefits and preparation tips, making it a valuable resource for anyone interested in early childhood nutrition.

No matter where you fall in the spectrum of parenting or caregiving, *100 Foods Before One Year* is your indispensable companion, guiding you with expertise and support as you embark on this exciting chapter of your baby's development.

WHY 100 FOODS BY ONE?

In the world of baby nutrition and weaning, we often hear the saying, "Food before one is just for fun." While there's truth to the idea that a baby's primary source of nutrition remains breast milk or formula during the first year of life, the introduction of solid foods is a crucial developmental milestone. It's the start of a beautiful relationship between your child and the diverse world of flavors and textures that food has to offer.

Introducing your baby to a variety of 100 different foods by their first birthday is not a strict requirement, but it's a valuable goal for several important reasons.

Nutritional Diversity: Different foods offer a wide range of essential nutrients. By exposing your baby to 100 different foods, you increase the likelihood that they receive a diverse array of vitamins, minerals, and other nutrients crucial for their growth and development.

Palate Development: Early exposure to various flavors and textures helps develop your baby's palate. It can make them more open to trying new foods later in life, potentially reducing picky eating habits.

Allergy Prevention: Gradually introducing a variety of foods may reduce the risk of developing food allergies. It's important to follow guidelines for introducing common allergens safely.

Health and Wellness: A diverse diet promotes overall health and wellness. It can contribute to a balanced diet and potentially reduce the risk of nutritional deficiencies.

Culinary Adventure: Food is not only about nutrition but also about cultural and sensory experiences. Exploring 100 different foods can be an exciting culinary adventure for your baby, helping them appreciate the rich tapestry of flavors and cuisines in the world.

Remember that this goal is not meant to be rigid, and it's crucial to prioritize your baby's comfort and nutritional needs. Always consult with a pediatrician or healthcare provider for guidance on your baby's specific dietary requirements, especially if you have concerns about allergies or other health conditions. The primary goal is to ensure your baby receives balanced nutrition and enjoys a positive relationship with food.

ALLERGENS

HOW TO INTRODUCE ALLERGENS

Introducing allergens to babies is an important aspect of their early nutrition. It helps reduce the risk of food allergies and desensitizes their immune system in a controlled manner. Here's a general guideline on how to introduce allergens and what it means:

Timing: Introduce allergenic foods when your baby is ready for solids, typically around 6 months of age. Always consult with your pediatrician to ensure it's the right time for your child.

Start with Single Foods: Introduce allergenic foods one at a time and in a simple, puréed form. This allows you to identify any potential allergic reactions more easily. Common allergenic foods include peanuts, tree nuts, eggs, dairy, soy, wheat, fish, and shellfish.

Gradual Introduction: Offer a small amount of the allergenic food and observe your baby closely for any signs of an allergic reaction. Common symptoms include hives, swelling, vomiting, diarrhea, or breathing difficulties. These reactions are typically immediate but can occur within two hours of ingestion.

Wait Between Introductions: Wait several days before introducing another allergenic food. This gap helps isolate the source of any potential allergic reactions. If your baby tolerates a particular food without any issues, you can continue to include it in their diet.

Early and Regular Exposure: Research suggests that introducing allergenic foods early and regularly (at least 2—3 times per week) can help reduce the risk of allergies. However, it's crucial to consult with your pediatrician, especially if your baby has a family history of allergies.

Consult a Pediatrician: If your baby has a known family history of food allergies or other risk factors, it's essential to discuss an allergen introduction plan with your pediatrician. They may recommend allergy testing or a specific introduction schedule.

Be Prepared: In case of a severe allergic reaction (anaphylaxis), have an epinephrine auto-injector (e.g., EpiPen) on hand, as prescribed by your pediatrician. Familiarize yourself with how to use it.

Monitor and Adapt: Pay attention to your baby's response to allergenic foods. If they show signs of an allergic reaction, stop offering that food and consult a healthcare professional immediately.

Remember that food allergies can be serious, but early and careful introduction of allergenic foods can be a proactive step in reducing the risk. Always prioritize your baby's safety and consult with your healthcare provider to create a personalized plan that considers your child's specific needs and risk factors.

WHAT ALLERGENS EXIST?

Common food allergens are substances that can trigger allergic reactions when ingested by individuals with specific sensitivities or allergies. Here are some common food allergens and brief descriptions of each:

Peanuts: Peanuts are legumes, not true nuts. They are a prevalent allergen and can cause severe allergic reactions. Peanut allergies tend to be lifelong and are rarely outgrown.

Tree Nuts: Tree nuts include almonds, walnuts, cashews, pistachios, and others. Allergies to tree nuts can vary in severity and may also be lifelong.

Eggs: Egg allergies are common in children but are often outgrown. The proteins in both the egg white and yolk can trigger allergic reactions.

Dairy: Dairy allergies involve a reaction to proteins found in milk, such as casein and whey. These allergies can affect children and adults and may cause digestive or skin reactions.

Soy: Soybeans and soy products can be allergenic. Soy allergies can manifest as skin reactions, digestive issues, or respiratory symptoms.

Wheat: Wheat contains gluten, which can trigger allergic reactions, particularly in individuals with wheat allergy or celiac disease. Wheat allergy is different from gluten sensitivity or celiac disease.

Fish: Allergic reactions to fish can be severe, and they often develop in adulthood. Common fish allergens include salmon, tuna, and cod.

Shellfish: Shellfish allergies can be divided into two categories: crustaceans (e.g., shrimp, crab, lobster) and mollusks (e.g., clams, mussels, oysters). Reactions to shellfish can be severe and are typically lifelong.

Sesame: Sesame allergy has become more recognized in recent years. It can cause allergic reactions similar to other food allergies, including skin rashes and respiratory symptoms.

Mustard: Mustard allergies are less common but can trigger allergic reactions when consumed. Mustard seeds and products containing mustard should be avoided by those with this allergy.

It's important to note that food allergies can vary in severity, with some individuals experiencing mild symptoms, while others may have life-threatening reactions (anaphylaxis). Allergies can also change over time, so it's essential to consult with a healthcare professional for proper diagnosis and management if you suspect a food allergy in yourself or your child.

WHAT TO DO IF YOUR BABY HAS AN ALLERGIC REACTION

If your baby has an allergic reaction, it's crucial to act quickly and follow these steps:

Stay Calm: Remain as calm as possible to provide the best care for your baby.

Assess the Symptoms: Observe your baby's symptoms. Allergic reactions can vary in severity but may include hives, swelling (especially of the face, lips, or tongue), difficulty breathing, coughing, wheezing, vomiting, diarrhea, or a change in behavior.

Call 911 (or Emergency Services): If your baby is experiencing severe symptoms, such as difficulty breathing, swelling of the throat, or a loss of consciousness, call 911 or your local emergency services immediately. Time is of the essence in such situations.

Lay Your Baby Down: If your baby is conscious and experiencing milder symptoms, lay them down on their back. This can help with breathing and circulation.

Offer Comfort: Reassure your baby and provide comfort. Keep them as calm as possible.

Monitor Vital Signs: Continuously monitor your baby's vital signs, including their breathing, pulse, and consciousness. Be prepared to provide CPR if necessary.

Seek Medical Attention: Even if the symptoms seem to improve after using epinephrine or if they were initially mild, seek immediate medical attention. Allergic reactions can have delayed or recurring symptoms.

Inform Healthcare Professionals: When you arrive at the hospital or medical facility, inform the healthcare professionals about the allergic reaction, what caused it (if known), and any treatment you administered.

It's crucial to have an emergency action plan in place if your baby has known food allergies. This plan should include knowledge of allergenic foods, prescribed epinephrine, and instructions on how and when to use it. Additionally, consult with your child's pediatrician or an allergist to develop a comprehensive allergy management plan tailored to your baby's specific needs.

PURÉE VS. BABY-LED WEANING

PURÉE FEEDING

Texture: Purée feeding involves offering foods that are blended into a smooth, semi-liquid consistency, including fruits, vegetables, grains, and proteins.

Introduction: It's typically introduced as a baby's first solid foods, usually around 6 months, as babies show signs of readiness.

Spoon-Feeding: Parents or caregivers use a spoon to feed these purées to the baby, giving precise control over the food type and amount.

Advantages: Purées are easy for babies to swallow, less likely to pose choking hazards, and allow for controlled introduction of flavors and nutrients.

BABY-LED WEANING

Texture: In BLW, babies are offered appropriately sized, graspable pieces of regular family foods, with varying textures, encouraging self-feeding.

Introduction: BLW is introduced when the baby is ready for solid foods, typically around 6 months, emphasizing self-regulation and independence.

Self-Feeding: Babies grasp and feed themselves, promoting fine motor skills and a positive relationship with food.

Advantages: BLW exposes babies to various flavors and textures, fosters self-regulation, and can be convenient for parents, avoiding the need for purée preparation.

MIXTURE (COMBINATION FEEDING)

Flexible Approach: Combination feeding combines purées and soft, age-appropriate finger foods, adapting to the baby's preferences and readiness.

Variety: It provides a variety of textures and tastes, offering the benefits of both methods.

Example: Parents may introduce mashed sweet potatoes alongside small, soft avocado or banana pieces.

Personalized Choice: The choice between purée feeding, BLW, or a combination depends on parental preference, baby's readiness, and specific considerations like allergies.

CONSIDERATIONS

Safety: Ensure food preparation minimizes choking hazards, closely supervise meals, and be aware of potential allergens.

Nutritional Balance: Regardless of the method, provide a balanced diet meeting the baby's nutritional needs.

Combination: Some parents opt for a blend of purée feeding and BLW, capitalizing on both approaches.

Ultimately, the choice between purée feeding and baby-led weaning depends on personal preference, baby's readiness, and individual needs. Consult a pediatrician or healthcare professional for guidance, recognizing that each baby is unique, with varying needs and abilities.

SAFETY: GAGGING VS. CHOKING

Gagging and choking are two distinct but related safety concerns when feeding a baby. It's crucial for parents and caregivers to understand the difference between them:

GAGGING

Gagging is a natural reflex that helps protect a baby from choking. When a baby gags, it means that a foreign object or food has touched the back of their throat or triggered their gag reflex.

Gagging is a common occurrence during the early stages of introducing solids, especially with baby-led weaning, where babies are learning to manipulate and swallow solid foods.

When a baby gags, they may make retching or coughing sounds, and it may look like they are struggling to swallow. However, they are actively working to push the object or food forward, away from the airway.

Gagging during feeding is a normal part of a baby's learning process and should not be a cause for panic. It usually resolves on its own as the baby becomes more skilled at handling different textures of food.

CHOKING

Choking, on the other hand, is a life-threatening emergency where an object or piece of food becomes lodged in the baby's airway, blocking their ability to breathe.

Choking is characterized by the inability to cough, cry, or make any sound. The baby may appear panicked, turn blue or pale, and struggle to breathe.

In the case of choking, immediate action is required to dislodge the obstructing object. Techniques like back blows and chest thrusts (for infants) or the Heimlich maneuver (for older babies) should be used to clear the airway.

It's essential for parents and caregivers to be vigilant and knowledgeable about both gagging and choking when introducing solid foods to a baby.

SAFETY TIP

- Always supervise your baby during mealtime.
- Offer age-appropriate, soft, and safely prepared foods.
- Cut foods into small, manageable pieces to minimize the risk of choking.
- Be prepared and learn infant CPR and choking rescue techniques.
- Stay calm in the event of gagging or choking, and take appropriate action based on the situation.

Remember that while gagging is a normal part of a baby's learning process when transitioning to solids, choking is a serious and life-threatening emergency. Understanding the difference between the two and knowing how to respond can help ensure your baby's safety during mealtime.

FOOD LIST

Introducing a variety of foods to a baby is an excellent way to expand their palate and provide essential nutrients. Here's a list of 150 different foods that you can consider introducing to your baby as they progress in their solid food journey. Keep in mind that you should introduce these foods based on your baby's age, developmental readiness, and any specific dietary considerations or allergies:

Fruits:

1. Apples
2. Bananas
3. Pears
4. Peaches
5. Plums
6. Apricots
7. Cherries
8. Blueberries
9. Strawberries
10. Raspberries
11. Blackberries
12. Mango
13. Papaya
14. Kiwi
15. Watermelon
16. Cantaloupe
17. Honeydew melon
18. Oranges
19. Pineapple
20. Grapes
21. Cranberries
22. Avocado
23. Figs
24. Guava
25. Passion fruit

Vegetables:

26. Sweet potatoes
27. Carrots
28. Butternut squash
29. Zucchini
30. Peas
31. Green beans
32. Broccoli
33. Cauliflower
34. Spinach
35. Kale
36. Swiss chard
37. Bell peppers
38. Tomatoes
39. Cucumbers
40. Asparagus
41. Eggplant
42. Beets
43. Turnips
44. Rutabaga
45. Celery
46. Peppers
47. Potatoes
48. Parsnips
49. Radishes
50. Cabbage

Grains and Cereals:

51. Rice
52. Oatmeal
53. Barley
54. Quinoa
55. Millet
56. Couscous
57. Whole wheat pasta
58. Brown rice
59. Farro
60. Buckwheat
61. Bulgur
62. Amaranth
63. Teff
64. Whole wheat bread
65. Rice cakes
66. Whole grain waffles

Proteins:

67. Chicken
68. Turkey
69. Beef
70. Pork
71. Lamb
72. Salmon
73. Tuna
74. Cod
75. Tilapia
76. Whitefish
77. Shrimp
78. Tofu
79. Tempeh
80. Lentils

Dairy and Dairy Alternatives:

81. Plain yogurt
82. Greek yogurt
83. Cottage cheese
84. Ricotta cheese
85. Cheddar cheese
86. Mozzarella cheese
87. Cream cheese
88. Goat cheese
89. Almond yogurt
90. Coconut yogurt
91. Soy yogurt
92. Cashew cheese
93. Hemp milk
94. Almond milk
95. Coconut milk

Legumes:

96. Chickpeas
97. Black beans
98. Kidney beans
99. Pinto beans
100. Cannellini beans
101. Navy beans
102. Lima beans
103. Red lentils
104. Green lentils
105. Black-eyed peas
106. Split peas

Nuts and Seeds:

107. Almond butter
108. Peanut butter
109. Cashew butter
110. Sunflower seed butter
111. Pumpkin seeds
112. Chia seeds
113. Flaxseeds
114. Hemp seeds
115. Sesame seeds

Herbs and Spices:

116. Cinnamon
117. Nutmeg
118. Basil
119. Parsley
120. Dill
121. Oregano
122. Thyme
123. Coriander
124. Turmeric
125. Cumin
126. Paprika

Dips and Sauces:

127. Hummus
128. Guacamole
129. Salsa
130. Applesauce
131. Greek yogurt dip
132. Tomato sauce

Miscellaneous:

133. Eggs
134. Rice pudding
135. Bread pudding
136. Pancakes
137. Waffles
138. Tapioca pudding
139. Rice cereal
140. Couscous pudding

Beverages:

141. Water
142. Breast milk
143. Infant formula
144. 100% fruit juice

Treats:

145. Raisins
146. Dates
147. Fig Newtons
148. Apple slices
149. Banana chips
150. Freeze-dried fruits

Food Tracker

Food Tracker

Food 1/100: _____

Allergen: ◯ yes   ◯ no

Acceptance: ☺   ☺   ☹

Preparation: raw   steamed   boiled   baked

Purée or solid

Occurrences/dates: _____

Notes:

Food 2/100: _____

Allergen: ◯ yes   ◯ no

Acceptance: ☺   ☺   ☹

Preparation: raw   steamed   boiled   baked

Purée or solid

Occurrences/dates: _____

Notes:

Food Tracker

Food 3/100: _____

Allergen: ○ yes   ○ no

Acceptance: ☺   😐   ☹

Preparation: raw   steamed   boiled   baked

Purée or solid

Occurrences/dates: _____

Notes:

Food 4/100: _____

Allergen: ○ yes   ○ no

Acceptance: ☺   😐   ☹

Preparation: raw   steamed   boiled   baked

Purée or solid

Occurrences/dates: _____

Notes:

Food Tracker

Food 5/100: _____

Allergen: ○ yes   ○ no

Acceptance: ☺   ☹   ☹

Preparation: raw   steamed   boiled   baked

Purée or solid

Occurrences/dates: _____

Notes:

Food 6/100: _____

Allergen: ○ yes   ○ no

Acceptance: ☺   ☹   ☹

Preparation: raw   steamed   boiled   baked

Purée or solid

Occurrences/dates: _____

Notes:

Food Tracker

Food 7/100: _____

Allergen: ○ yes ○ no

Acceptance: ☺ ☺ ☹

Preparation: raw   steamed   boiled   baked

Purée or solid

Occurrences/dates: _____

Notes:

Food 8/100: _____

Allergen: ○ yes ○ no

Acceptance: ☺ ☺ ☹

Preparation: raw   steamed   boiled   baked

Purée or solid

Occurrences/dates: _____

Notes:

Food Tracker

Food 9/100: _____

Allergen:　　○ yes　　○ no

Acceptance:　☺　　☹　　☹

Preparation:　raw　　steamed　　boiled　　baked

Purée　or　solid

Occurrences/dates: _____

Notes:

Food 10/100: _____

Allergen:　　○ yes　　○ no

Acceptance:　☺　　☹　　☹

Preparation:　raw　　steamed　　boiled　　baked

Purée　or　solid

Occurrences/dates: _____

Notes:

Food Tracker

Food 11/100: _____

Allergen: ○ yes   ○ no

Acceptance: ☺   ☺   ☹

Preparation: raw   steamed   boiled   baked

Purée or solid

Occurrences/dates: _____

Notes:

Food 12/100: _____

Allergen: ○ yes   ○ no

Acceptance: ☺   ☺   ☹

Preparation: raw   steamed   boiled   baked

Purée or solid

Occurrences/dates: _____

Notes:

Food Tracker

Food 13/100: _____

Allergen: ○ yes   ○ no

Acceptance: ☺   😕   ☹

Preparation: raw   steamed   boiled   baked

Purée or solid

Occurrences/dates: _____

Notes:

Food 14/100: _____

Allergen: ○ yes   ○ no

Acceptance: ☺   😕   ☹

Preparation: raw   steamed   boiled   baked

Purée or solid

Occurrences/dates: _____

Notes:

Food Tracker

Food 15/100: _____

Allergen: ○ yes ○ no

Acceptance: ☺ 😐 ☹

Preparation: raw steamed boiled baked

Purée or solid

Occurrences/dates: _____

Notes:

Food 16/100: _____

Allergen: ○ yes ○ no

Acceptance: ☺ 😐 ☹

Preparation: raw steamed boiled baked

Purée or solid

Occurrences/dates: _____

Notes:

Food Tracker

Food 17/100: _____

Allergen:　　○ yes　　○ no

Acceptance:　☺　　☹　　☹

Preparation:　raw　　steamed　　boiled　　baked

Purée or solid

Occurrences/dates: _____

Notes:

Food 18/100: _____

Allergen:　　○ yes　　○ no

Acceptance:　☺　　☹　　☹

Preparation:　raw　　steamed　　boiled　　baked

Purée or solid

Occurrences/dates: _____

Notes:

Food Tracker

Food 19/100: _____   Notes:

Allergen: ◯ yes   ◯ no

Acceptance: ☺   ☹   ☹

Preparation: raw   steamed   boiled   baked

Purée or solid

Occurrences/dates: _____

Food 20/100: _____   Notes:

Allergen: ◯ yes   ◯ no

Acceptance: ☺   ☹   ☹

Preparation: raw   steamed   boiled   baked

Purée or solid

Occurrences/dates: _____

Food Tracker

Food 21/100: _____

Allergen: ○ yes ○ no

Acceptance: ☺ ☹ ☹

Preparation: raw   steamed   boiled   baked

Purée or solid

Occurrences/dates: _____

Notes:

Food 22/100: _____

Allergen: ○ yes ○ no

Acceptance: ☺ ☹ ☹

Preparation: raw   steamed   boiled   baked

Purée or solid

Occurrences/dates: _____

Notes:

Food Tracker

Food 23/100: _____

Allergen: ○ yes   ○ no

Acceptance: ☺   ☺   ☹

Preparation: raw   steamed   boiled   baked

Purée or solid

Occurrences/dates: _____

Notes:

Food 24/100: _____

Allergen: ○ yes   ○ no

Acceptance: ☺   ☺   ☹

Preparation: raw   steamed   boiled   baked

Purée or solid

Occurrences/dates: _____

Notes:

Food Tracker

Food 25/100: _____

Allergen: ○ yes ○ no

Acceptance: ☺ 😐 ☹

Preparation: raw steamed boiled baked

Purée or solid

Occurrences/dates: _____

Notes:

Food 26/100: _____

Allergen: ○ yes ○ no

Acceptance: ☺ 😐 ☹

Preparation: raw steamed boiled baked

Purée or solid

Occurrences/dates: _____

Notes:

Food Tracker

Food 27/100: _____

Allergen: ○ yes   ○ no

Acceptance: ☺   😐   ☹

Preparation: raw   steamed   boiled   baked

Purée or solid

Occurrences/dates: _____

Notes:

Food 28/100: _____

Allergen: ○ yes   ○ no

Acceptance: ☺   😐   ☹

Preparation: raw   steamed   boiled   baked

Purée or solid

Occurrences/dates: _____

Notes:

Food Tracker

Food 29/100: _____

Allergen: ○ yes   ○ no

Acceptance: ☺   😐   ☹

Preparation: raw   steamed   boiled   baked

Purée or solid

Occurrences/dates: _____

Notes:

Food 30/100: _____

Allergen: ○ yes   ○ no

Acceptance: ☺   😐   ☹

Preparation: raw   steamed   boiled   baked

Purée or solid

Occurrences/dates: _____

Notes:

Food Tracker

Food 31/100: _____

Notes:

Allergen:　　○ yes　　○ no

Acceptance:　☺　　☹　　☹

Preparation:　raw　　steamed　　boiled　　baked

Purée or solid

Occurrences/dates: _____

Food 32/100: _____

Notes:

Allergen:　　○ yes　　○ no

Acceptance:　☺　　☹　　☹

Preparation:　raw　　steamed　　boiled　　baked

Purée or solid

Occurrences/dates: _____

Food Tracker

Food 33/100: _____

Allergen: ◯ yes ◯ no

Acceptance: ☺ ☺ ☹

Preparation: raw   steamed   boiled   baked

Purée or solid

Occurrences/dates: _____

Notes:

Food 34/100: _____

Allergen: ◯ yes ◯ no

Acceptance: ☺ ☺ ☹

Preparation: raw   steamed   boiled   baked

Purée or solid

Occurrences/dates: _____

Notes:

Food Tracker

Food 35/100: _____

Allergen: ◯ yes   ◯ no

Acceptance: ☺   😐   ☹

Preparation: raw   steamed   boiled   baked

Purée or solid

Occurrences/dates: _____

Notes:

Food 36/100: _____

Allergen: ◯ yes   ◯ no

Acceptance: ☺   😐   ☹

Preparation: raw   steamed   boiled   baked

Purée or solid

Occurrences/dates: _____

Notes:

Food Tracker

Food 37/100: _____

Allergen: ○ yes   ○ no

Acceptance: ☺   😐   ☹

Preparation: raw   steamed   boiled   baked

Purée or solid

Occurrences/dates: _____

Notes:

Food 38/100: _____

Allergen: ○ yes   ○ no

Acceptance: ☺   😐   ☹

Preparation: raw   steamed   boiled   baked

Purée or solid

Occurrences/dates: _____

Notes:

Food Tracker

Food 39/100: _____

Allergen: ○ yes   ○ no

Acceptance: ☺   😐   ☹

Preparation: raw   steamed   boiled   baked

Purée or solid

Occurrences/dates: _____

Notes:

Food 40/100: _____

Allergen: ○ yes   ○ no

Acceptance: ☺   😐   ☹

Preparation: raw   steamed   boiled   baked

Purée or solid

Occurrences/dates: _____

Notes:

Food Tracker

Food 41/100: _____

Allergen: ◯ yes   ◯ no

Acceptance: ☺   😐   ☹

Preparation: raw   steamed   boiled   baked

Purée or solid

Occurrences/dates: _____

Notes:

Food 42/100: _____

Allergen: ◯ yes   ◯ no

Acceptance: ☺   😐   ☹

Preparation: raw   steamed   boiled   baked

Purée or solid

Occurrences/dates: _____

Notes:

Food Tracker

Food 43/100: _____

Allergen:　　◯ yes　　◯ no

Acceptance:　☺　　☺　　☹

Preparation:　raw　steamed　boiled　baked

Purée or solid

Occurrences/dates: _____

Notes:

Food 44/100: _____

Allergen:　　◯ yes　　◯ no

Acceptance:　☺　　☺　　☹

Preparation:　raw　steamed　boiled　baked

Purée or solid

Occurrences/dates: _____

Notes:

Food Tracker

Food 45/100: _____

Allergen: ○ yes   ○ no

Acceptance: ☺   ☹   ☹

Preparation: raw   steamed   boiled   baked

Purée or solid

Occurrences/dates: _____

Notes:

Food 46/100: _____

Allergen: ○ yes   ○ no

Acceptance: ☺   ☹   ☹

Preparation: raw   steamed   boiled   baked

Purée or solid

Occurrences/dates: _____

Notes:

Food Tracker

Food 47/100: _____

Allergen: ○ yes   ○ no

Acceptance: ☺   ☺   ☹

Preparation: raw   steamed   boiled   baked

Purée or solid

Occurrences/dates: _____

Notes:

Food 48/100: _____

Allergen: ○ yes   ○ no

Acceptance: ☺   ☺   ☹

Preparation: raw   steamed   boiled   baked

Purée or solid

Occurrences/dates: _____

Notes:

Food Tracker

Food 49/100: _____

Allergen: ○ yes ○ no

Acceptance: ☺ 😐 ☹

Preparation: raw steamed boiled baked

Purée or solid

Occurrences/dates: _____

Notes:

Food 50/100: _____

Allergen: ○ yes ○ no

Acceptance: ☺ 😐 ☹

Preparation: raw steamed boiled baked

Purée or solid

Occurrences/dates: _____

Notes:

Food Tracker

Food 51/100: _____

Notes:

Allergen: ○ yes ○ no

Acceptance: ☺ ☹ ☹

Preparation: raw   steamed   boiled   baked

Purée or solid

Occurrences/dates: _____

Food 52/100: _____

Notes:

Allergen: ○ yes ○ no

Acceptance: ☺ ☹ ☹

Preparation: raw   steamed   boiled   baked

Purée or solid

Occurrences/dates: _____

Food Tracker

Food 53/100: _____

Allergen: ○ yes   ○ no

Acceptance: ☺   ☹   ☹

Preparation: raw   steamed   boiled   baked

Purée or solid

Occurrences/dates: _____

Notes:

Food 54/100: _____

Allergen: ○ yes   ○ no

Acceptance: ☺   ☹   ☹

Preparation: raw   steamed   boiled   baked

Purée or solid

Occurrences/dates: _____

Notes:

Food Tracker

Food 55/100: _____

Allergen: ○ yes   ○ no

Acceptance: ☺   ☺   ☹

Preparation: raw   steamed   boiled   baked

Purée or solid

Occurrences/dates: _____

Notes:

Food 56/100: _____

Allergen: ○ yes   ○ no

Acceptance: ☺   ☺   ☹

Preparation: raw   steamed   boiled   baked

Purée or solid

Occurrences/dates: _____

Notes:

Food Tracker

Food 57/100: _____

Allergen: ◯ yes ◯ no

Acceptance: ☺ ☺ ☹

Preparation: raw steamed boiled baked

Purée or solid

Occurrences/dates: _____

Notes:

Food 58/100: _____

Allergen: ◯ yes ◯ no

Acceptance: ☺ ☺ ☹

Preparation: raw steamed boiled baked

Purée or solid

Occurrences/dates: _____

Notes:

Food Tracker

Food 59/100: _____   Notes:

Allergen: ○ yes   ○ no

Acceptance: ☺ ☺ ☹

Preparation: raw   steamed   boiled   baked

Purée or solid

Occurrences/dates: _____

Food 60/100: _____   Notes:

Allergen: ○ yes   ○ no

Acceptance: ☺ ☺ ☹

Preparation: raw   steamed   boiled   baked

Purée or solid

Occurrences/dates: _____

Food Tracker

Food 61/100: _____

Allergen: ○ yes ○ no

Acceptance: ☺ 😐 ☹

Preparation: raw steamed boiled baked

Purée or solid

Occurrences/dates: _____

Notes:

Food 62/100: _____

Allergen: ○ yes ○ no

Acceptance: ☺ 😐 ☹

Preparation: raw steamed boiled baked

Purée or solid

Occurrences/dates: _____

Notes:

Food Tracker

Food 63/100: _____

Allergen: ○ yes ○ no

Acceptance: ☺ ☺ ☹

Preparation: raw   steamed   boiled   baked

Purée or solid

Occurrences/dates: _____

Notes:

Food 64/100: _____

Allergen: ○ yes ○ no

Acceptance: ☺ ☺ ☹

Preparation: raw   steamed   boiled   baked

Purée or solid

Occurrences/dates: _____

Notes:

Food Tracker

Food 65/100: _____

Allergen:　　○ yes　　○ no

Acceptance:　☺　　☹　　☹

Preparation:　raw　steamed　boiled　baked

Purée　or　solid

Occurrences/dates: _____

Notes:

Food 66/100: _____

Allergen:　　○ yes　　○ no

Acceptance:　☺　　☹　　☹

Preparation:　raw　steamed　boiled　baked

Purée　or　solid

Occurrences/dates: _____

Notes:

Food Tracker

Food 67/100: _____

Allergen: ○ yes   ○ no

Acceptance: ☺   😐   ☹

Preparation: raw   steamed   boiled   baked

Purée or solid

Occurrences/dates: _____

Notes:

Food 68/100: _____

Allergen: ○ yes   ○ no

Acceptance: ☺   😐   ☹

Preparation: raw   steamed   boiled   baked

Purée or solid

Occurrences/dates: _____

Notes:

Food Tracker

Food 69/100: _____

Allergen: ○ yes   ○ no

Acceptance: ☺   ☺   ☹

Preparation: raw   steamed   boiled   baked

Purée or solid

Occurrences/dates: _____

Notes:

Food 70/100: _____

Allergen: ○ yes   ○ no

Acceptance: ☺   ☺   ☹

Preparation: raw   steamed   boiled   baked

Purée or solid

Occurrences/dates: _____

Notes:

Food Tracker

Food 71/100: _____

Allergen: ◯ yes ◯ no

Acceptance: ☺ 😐 ☹

Preparation: raw   steamed   boiled   baked

Purée or solid

Occurrences/dates: _____

Notes:

Food 72/100: _____

Allergen: ◯ yes ◯ no

Acceptance: ☺ 😐 ☹

Preparation: raw   steamed   boiled   baked

Purée or solid

Occurrences/dates: _____

Notes:

Food Tracker

Food 73/100: _____

Allergen: ○ yes ○ no

Acceptance: ☺ ☺ ☹

Preparation: raw steamed boiled baked

Purée or solid

Occurrences/dates: _____

Notes:

Food 74/100: _____

Allergen: ○ yes ○ no

Acceptance: ☺ ☺ ☹

Preparation: raw steamed boiled baked

Purée or solid

Occurrences/dates: _____

Notes:

Food Tracker

Food 75/100: _____   Notes:

Allergen: ○ yes   ○ no

Acceptance: ☺ ☹ ☹

Preparation: raw   steamed   boiled   baked

Purée or solid

Occurrences/dates: _____

Food 76/100: _____   Notes:

Allergen: ○ yes   ○ no

Acceptance: ☺ ☹ ☹

Preparation: raw   steamed   boiled   baked

Purée or solid

Occurrences/dates: _____

Food Tracker

Food 77/100: _____ Notes:

Allergen: ◯ yes ◯ no

Acceptance: ☺ ☺ ☹

Preparation: raw steamed boiled baked

Purée or solid

Occurrences/dates: _____

Food 78/100: _____ Notes:

Allergen: ◯ yes ◯ no

Acceptance: ☺ ☺ ☹

Preparation: raw steamed boiled baked

Purée or solid

Occurrences/dates: _____

Food Tracker

Food 79/100: _____

Allergen: ○ yes ○ no

Acceptance: ☺ ☹ ☹

Preparation: raw   steamed   boiled   baked

Purée or solid

Occurrences/dates: _____

Notes:

Food 80/100: _____

Allergen: ○ yes ○ no

Acceptance: ☺ ☹ ☹

Preparation: raw   steamed   boiled   baked

Purée or solid

Occurrences/dates: _____

Notes:

Food Tracker

Food 81/100: _____

Allergen: ○ yes   ○ no

Acceptance: ☺   😐   ☹

Preparation: raw   steamed   boiled   baked

Purée or solid

Occurrences/dates: _____

Notes:

Food 82/100: _____

Allergen: ○ yes   ○ no

Acceptance: ☺   😐   ☹

Preparation: raw   steamed   boiled   baked

Purée or solid

Occurrences/dates: _____

Notes:

Food Tracker

Food 83/100: _____   Notes:

Allergen: ○ yes   ○ no

Acceptance: ☺   😐   ☹

Preparation: raw   steamed   boiled   baked

Purée or solid

Occurrences/dates: _____

Food 84/100: _____   Notes:

Allergen: ○ yes   ○ no

Acceptance: ☺   😐   ☹

Preparation: raw   steamed   boiled   baked

Purée or solid

Occurrences/dates: _____

Food Tracker

Food 85/100: _____

Allergen: ○ yes ○ no

Acceptance: ☺ ☹ ☹

Preparation: raw steamed boiled baked

Purée or solid

Occurrences/dates: _____

Notes:

Food 86/100: _____

Allergen: ○ yes ○ no

Acceptance: ☺ ☹ ☹

Preparation: raw steamed boiled baked

Purée or solid

Occurrences/dates: _____

Notes:

Food Tracker

Food 87/100: _____

Allergen: ○ yes   ○ no

Acceptance: ☺   ☺   ☹

Preparation: raw   steamed   boiled   baked

Purée or solid

Occurrences/dates: _____

Notes:

Food 88/100: _____

Allergen: ○ yes   ○ no

Acceptance: ☺   ☺   ☹

Preparation: raw   steamed   boiled   baked

Purée or solid

Occurrences/dates: _____

Notes:

Food Tracker

Food 89/100: _____

Allergen: ○ yes   ○ no

Acceptance: ☺   ☺   ☹

Preparation: raw   steamed   boiled   baked

Purée or solid

Occurrences/dates: _____

Notes:

Food 90/100: _____

Allergen: ○ yes   ○ no

Acceptance: ☺   ☺   ☹

Preparation: raw   steamed   boiled   baked

Purée or solid

Occurrences/dates: _____

Notes:

Food Tracker

Food 91/100: _____   Notes:

Allergen: ○ yes   ○ no

Acceptance: ☺   😐   ☹

Preparation: raw   steamed   boiled   baked

Purée or solid

Occurrences/dates: _____

Food 92/100: _____   Notes:

Allergen: ○ yes   ○ no

Acceptance: ☺   😐   ☹

Preparation: raw   steamed   boiled   baked

Purée or solid

Occurrences/dates: _____

Food Tracker

Food 93/100: _____

Allergen: ○ yes ○ no

Acceptance: ☺ ☹ ☹

Preparation: raw steamed boiled baked

Purée or solid

Occurrences/dates: _____

Notes:

Food 94/100: _____

Allergen: ○ yes ○ no

Acceptance: ☺ ☹ ☹

Preparation: raw steamed boiled baked

Purée or solid

Occurrences/dates: _____

Notes:

Food Tracker

Food 95/100: _____

Allergen: ○ yes   ○ no

Acceptance: ☺   ☻   ☹

Preparation: raw   steamed   boiled   baked

Purée or solid

Occurrences/dates: _____

Notes:

Food 96/100: _____

Allergen: ○ yes   ○ no

Acceptance: ☺   ☻   ☹

Preparation: raw   steamed   boiled   baked

Purée or solid

Occurrences/dates: _____

Notes:

Food Tracker

Food 97/100: _____

Allergen: ◯ yes ◯ no

Acceptance: ☺ 😕 ☹

Preparation: raw steamed boiled baked

Purée or solid

Occurrences/dates: _____

Notes:

Food 98/100: _____

Allergen: ◯ yes ◯ no

Acceptance: ☺ 😕 ☹

Preparation: raw steamed boiled baked

Purée or solid

Occurrences/dates: _____

Notes:

Food Tracker

Food 99/100: _____   Notes:

Allergen: ◯ yes   ◯ no

Acceptance: ☺   😐   ☹

Preparation: raw   steamed   boiled   baked

Purée or solid

Occurrences/dates: _____

Food 100/100: _____   Notes:

Allergen: ◯ yes   ◯ no

Acceptance: ☺   😐   ☹

Preparation: raw   steamed   boiled   baked

Purée or solid

Occurrences/dates: _____

ALLERGEN LIST

DATE	FOOD	REACTION

ALLERGEN LIST

DATE	FOOD	REACTION

ALLERGEN LIST

DATE	FOOD	REACTION